1

DISCLAIMER

This book's content is only intended for general informative purposes. At the time of writing, the author has taken every precaution to guarantee that the material is correct and current. Nevertheless, the author disclaims all explicit and implicit representations and guarantees about the availability, appropriateness, correctness, completeness, and usefulness of the material on these pages.

Since the author is not a licensed medical practitioner, the material in this book shouldn't be interpreted as medical advice. Before making any modifications to their diet, exercise regimen, or medical treatment, readers are urged to speak with a licensed healthcare provider.

Moreover, the author has no connection to any of the businesses, organizations, or people that are discussed in this book. Any mentions of goods, services, businesses, or people are purely informative and do not indicate endorsement or suggestion.

This book's content is entirely dependent on the author's expertise, study, and comprehension of the topic. Despite having taken reasonable care to offer correct information, the author disclaims all liability for any mistakes or omissions in the material as well as for any losses, harm, or damages resulting from using the information.

It is recommended that readers use their own judgment and discretion when applying the knowledge in this book to their own situations. The use or implementation of any material in this book may result in unfavorable repercussions, directly or indirectly, for which the author assumes no liability.

By reading this book, you agree to release and hold the author harmless from any claims, losses, liabilities, costs, or expenditures resulting from or related to the use of the information you get from it.

Table of Contents

ABOUT THE BOOK

"Hernia" is more than simply a medical book; it's a thorough manual that gives readers the confidence to comprehend, treat, and negotiate the complexity of hernias. This book is an invaluable resource for anybody afflicted by hernias or looking to avoid them, with chapters carefully designed to cover all elements of hernia care, from understanding the problem to living with it and researching future therapies.

Establishing the basics, Chapter 1 gives a concise overview of hernias, explaining their many kinds, causes, and risk factors. Readers learn vital information about the nature and causes of this widespread yet often misdiagnosed illness by deciphering it.

In Chapter 2, readers gain the ability to detect the telltale signs and symptoms of hernias, enabling them to determine when seeking medical help is necessary and comprehend the possible consequences of treating hernias without treatment. This information may save lives by enabling immediate action and averting further health issues.

In Chapter 3, the diagnostic procedure is explored in detail, providing readers with an understanding of the several tests and exams that are used to diagnose hernias. People may approach their healthcare experience with better clarity and confidence if they understand how diagnoses are made.

Chapter 4 then delves into treatment alternatives, ranging from conservative measures like lifestyle adjustments and cautious waiting to more drastic measures like surgical treatments. Readers are empowered to make selections based on their circumstances, preferences, and health objectives by being presented with a variety of options.

In Chapter 5, readers get vital advice on what to anticipate before, during, and after the treatment, including possible risks and problems. This information is especially helpful as readers get ready for surgery. This knowledge reduces fears and encourages the best possible results by empowering people to feel prepared and in control.

With an emphasis on the recuperation process, Chapter 6 provides helpful guidance on managing pain, returning to everyday activities, and post-operative care. People may minimize setbacks and confidently traverse the recovery route by adhering to these suggestions.

Readers may learn about probable post-surgery issues and recurrences in Chapter 7, as well as measures to reduce risks and know when to seek medical assistance. People are empowered to take control of their health and well-being outside of the operation room with this proactive approach.

The comprehensive features of living with a hernia are covered in Chapter 8, including coping mechanisms, food advice, psychological effects, and avenues for assistance. This chapter discusses the mental, emotional, and social aspects of managing a hernia and encourages resilience and overall well-being.

The particular concerns for hernias in certain populations—such as newborns, toddlers, pregnant women, and elderly adults—are highlighted in Chapter 9. The book makes sure that the material is inclusive and relevant to a wide range of readers by customizing it for certain demographics.

Chapter 10 provides a last look at the care of hernias in the future by examining new therapies, developments in the field, and opportunities for patient advocacy and support. By keeping up to date on emerging trends and advances, readers may actively participate in their healthcare process and help progress the treatment of hernias.

To put it simply, "Hernia" is more than just a book— it's a source of information, strength, and hope for those who are dealing with hernias and those who care about their health. This book is a valuable resource for anybody affected by hernias because of its abundance of knowledge, helpful advice, and optimistic outlook. It provides a clear path to better health in the future.

CHAPTER 1

Introduction To Hernias

Despite their frightening name, hernias are rather common, and knowing what they are may ease a lot of anxiety. A hernia happens when fat or an organ pushes through a weak place in the surrounding connective tissue or muscle, bulging the surrounding area. The fundamental concept is to visualize a balloon pushing through a weak area in a tire.

What Is A Hernia?

Usually an obvious lump or protrusion, a hernia is also associated with pain or discomfort, particularly when moving heavy things, coughing, or straining during bowel motions. This bulge occurs when tissue or internal organs push through a weak spot in the muscle or connective tissue, which usually occurs in the abdomen wall.

Types Of Hernias (Inguinal, Femoral, Umbilical, Etc.)

There are many varieties of hernias, each with unique traits and locations inside the body. The most typical kinds consist of:

• **Inguinal Hernia:** This is the most common kind, which happens when an intestinal segment pokes through the lower abdominal wall's inguinal canal.

• **Femoral Hernia:** Via the femoral canal, this condition is similar to an inguinal hernia but occurs further down, close to the groin. These are more typical in females.

• **Umbilical Hernia:** This kind is characterized by a protrusion close to the belly button, where a portion of the intestine or fatty tissue protrudes through a weak point in the abdominal wall.

• **Incisional hernia:** This kind appears where a prior surgical incision was made, either from tissue pushing through the scar or weakening muscles.

• **Hiatal Hernia:** Not to be confused with the other types, this one happens when the upper portion of the stomach pushes through the diaphragm and into the chest cavity, resulting in symptoms such as acid reflux.

Causes And Risk Factors

Prevention and early identification of hernias may be aided by knowledge of the causes and risk factors. Among the frequent reasons and danger signs are:

• **Abdominal wall weakness:** This may be inherited (existing from birth) or develop over time as a result of age, trauma, or strain.

- **Strain and Pressure:** Pregnancy, hard lifting, chronic coughing, obesity, and other circumstances that raise pressure in the abdominal cavity may all lead to hernias.

- **Genetics:** Some people are predisposed to weak abdominal muscles or connective tissue, which increases their risk of hernias.

- **Gender:** Men are more likely than women to suffer from inguinal hernias, whilst women are more likely to suffer from femoral hernias.

- **Age:** As individuals age, their muscles and connective tissue gradually weaken, which increases the incidence of hernias.

- **Chronic Constipation or Straining:** By placing extra pressure on the abdominal wall, conditions that need repeated straining during bowel movements might raise the risk of hernias.

CHAPTER 2

Signs And Symptoms

Common Symptoms Of Hernias

The range of symptoms associated with hernias varies according to the kind and extent of the hernia. Usually in the abdominal or groin region, a prominent lump or protrusion is one of the most prevalent symptoms. Lying down may cause this bulge to vanish, but standing or exerting yourself may make it more noticeable. It sometimes comes with pain or discomfort, especially when moving large things or engaging in physical activities.

A dull pain or a heavy sensation in the afflicted region is another typical symptom. This ache or feeling may become worse throughout the day or after extended standing or sitting. A scorching or shooting pain at the location of the hernia may also be experienced by some individuals, particularly while coughing, sneezing, or straining during bowel motions.

Furthermore, gastrointestinal symptoms like nausea, vomiting, or acid reflux may be brought on by hernias, especially if the hernia affects the digestive organs and is situated in the abdominal wall. Urinary urgency or frequency, difficulties passing stool or urine, and even urinary retention may sometimes result from hernias if they compress surrounding tissues.

It's crucial to remember that not all hernias, particularly in the early stages, generate symptoms. Unintentionally, some hernias may be found during a physical examination or imaging procedure for a different issue. However, it's critical to get medical attention right away if you have any persistent symptoms that could point to a hernia.

When To Seek Medical Attention

For a hernia to be diagnosed and treated promptly, it is important to know when to seek medical help. Even while not every hernia has to be treated right once, several symptoms and indicators call for a quick assessment by a medical expert.

Make an appointment with your health care physician or a hernia specialist if you discover a new or growing lump or bulge in your belly or groin region, particularly if it causes pain, discomfort, or changes in your bowel or urine habits. In a similar vein, get medical help right once if you have a known hernia that becomes unexpectedly sensitive, painful, or irreducible (cannot be put back in).

In addition, symptoms including fever, nausea, vomiting, and bowel obstructions such as severe stomach discomfort, bloating, constipation, or difficulty passing gas should be promptly evaluated by a doctor. These signs might point to a hernia complication like strangling or imprisonment, which calls for emergency medical attention to stop tissue damage and perhaps fatal consequences.

Generally speaking, it's best to err on the side of caution and seek examination from a trained healthcare expert if you're not sure if your symptoms deserve medical treatment. Ignoring symptoms or putting off treatment might make the situation worse and perhaps need more invasive surgery later on.

Complications Of Untreated Hernias

If a hernia is left untreated, it may result in several consequences, some of which are potentially fatal. The most dangerous side effect is strangling, in which an intestinal loop becomes stuck in the hernia sac and stops receiving blood. This may cause the confined intestine to become necrotic (tissue dead) and ischemia (lack of blood flow), resulting in a medical emergency that calls for urgent surgery to stop sepsis (a potentially fatal infection) and systemic organ failure.

Incarceration, in which the hernia becomes irreducible or imprisoned outside the abdominal cavity, is another possible consequence. If left untreated, this may create chronic pain, swelling, and discomfort at the hernia site and raise the risk of strangulation. Untreated hernias may sometimes enlarge over time, resulting in more severe symptoms and making surgical treatment more difficult.

Chronic hernias that go untreated may also result in consequences like bowel obstruction, which is a blockage in the herniated intestine that prevents gas and feces from passing through. To release the blockage and return to normal bowel function, this may cause excruciating abdominal discomfort, distention, nausea, vomiting, and dehydration. Emergency medical attention may be necessary.

In conclusion, even though not all hernias need to be treated right away, it's important to keep a careful eye on your symptoms and visit a doctor if you notice any worrying symptoms or consequences. For those who have hernias, early detection and treatment may help avoid major problems and enhance results.

CHAPTER 3

Diagnosis

Physical Examination

A comprehensive physical examination performed by a medical practitioner is a crucial step in the diagnosis of a hernia. The doctor will usually inquire about your medical history and any current symptoms during this evaluation. After that, they will do a physical examination, which often entails looking at the afflicted region and feeling for any odd lumps or bulges. For instance, if you have an inguinal hernia, your doctor would ask you to cough or strain as they feel for any protrusions in your groin region.

The physician may also do examinations on other body areas to look for indications of complications or associated diseases.

For example, they might measure the abdominal muscles' strength and look for any indications of intestinal blockage.

Imaging Tests (Ultrasound, CT Scan, MRI)

To determine the severity of a hernia and confirm its existence, more imaging tests could be required in some situations. For this kind of imaging, CT, MRI, and ultrasound scans are often used.

High-frequency sound waves are used in ultrasound, a non-invasive imaging method, to provide finely detailed pictures of the inside of the body. Hernias are often visualized with it, especially those in the groin and abdomen. A tiny handheld device known as a transducer is gently dragged over the skin above the suspected hernia site during an ultrasound examination. It transmits sound waves that reflect off internal structures and produce pictures that are shown on a monitor.

Advanced imaging methods such as CT (computed tomography) and MRI (magnetic resonance imaging) may provide comprehensive cross-sectional pictures of the body. If the hernia is difficult to see with ultrasonography or if further assessment of the surrounding tissues is required, these tests could be prescribed. Whereas an MRI uses radio waves and a magnetic field to produce pictures without subjecting the patient to ionizing radiation, a CT scan uses X-rays and a computer to produce detailed images.

Diagnostic Procedures (Herniography)

To assess a hernia more thoroughly, it could be advised in certain circumstances to undergo extra diagnostic tests. Pornography is one such method that involves injecting a contrast dye into the abdominal cavity and then using X-rays or other imaging techniques to image the area.

The use of contrast dye during a herniography aids in highlighting the hernia and the surrounding structures, allowing a more thorough evaluation of the structure's size, location, and connection to adjacent organs. When the diagnosis cannot be made just from a physical examination and routine imaging studies, this method could be very helpful.

In general, a physical examination, imaging studies, and, if required, diagnostic techniques like herniography may assist medical professionals in correctly diagnosing a hernia and creating a customized treatment strategy for each patient. For individuals with hernias, attaining the best possible results and avoiding complications requires early identification and care.

CHAPTER 4

Treatment Options

Watchful Waiting

"Watch and wait," or "watchful waiting," is a treatment strategy for certain hernias, especially the tiny, asymptomatic ones. Instead of launching into surgery right once, medical professionals monitor the hernia's development over time, evaluating any modifications to its size, symptoms, or problems. This method is often used when the hernia is not significantly uncomfortable or interferes with day-to-day activities.

Patients are urged to remain aware of their hernia during careful waiting and to notify their healthcare physician right away if anything changes or becomes symptomatic. Check-ups are planned regularly to assess the condition of the hernia and make sure that the right treatment is done when needed. Imaging tests like an MRI or ultrasound may be necessary to determine the extent of the hernia and any related problems.

Waiting with caution has the benefit of preventing needless surgery for hernias that could stabilize or even go away on their own with time. However, to track the hernia's development and avoid any consequences, patients must follow their doctor's advice and make frequent follow-up consultations.

Lifestyle Changes And Prevention Tips

A few lifestyle adjustments may help control hernias and lower the chance of consequences. These adjustments often center on reducing variables that may raise intra-abdominal pressure, which may worsen or even cause hernias. Here are a few useful pointers:

1. **Keep Your Weight in Check:** Carrying too much weight may put a strain on your weaker abdominal

muscles and perhaps exacerbate hernias. It can also raise intra-abdominal pressure. A healthy weight may be attained and maintained with the support of a regular exercise program and a nutritious diet.

2. Steer clear of large Lifting: Hernias may be made worse by lifting large things, which can strain the abdominal muscles. Use safe lifting methods whenever you can, and stay away from heavy lifting completely if you have a hernia. When carrying big goods, think about utilizing assistive equipment or getting assistance from others.

3. Give Up Smoking: Smoking aggravates hernias and increases intra-abdominal pressure by causing coughing and other chronic respiratory problems. Giving up smoking may enhance general health and lower the chance of problems from hernias.

4. Handle Constipation: Excessive straining during bowel movements brought on by constipation may worsen hernias and raise intra-abdominal pressure. To successfully treat constipation, make sure you get enough fiber, remain hydrated, and think about over-the-counter medicines or lifestyle modifications.

5. Put on Supportive Garments: For some people, donning abdominal binders or hernia belts may provide extra comfort and support, especially while participating in physically demanding activities or jobs that might put stress on the abdominal muscles.

People may control their hernias and lower their risk of complications by adopting these lifestyle modifications. However, for tailored counsel and direction based on specific situations, it's imperative to speak with a healthcare expert.

Surgical Interventions (Open Repair, Laparoscopic Repair)

Surgical intervention may be required when hernias develop symptoms, dramatically grow, or offer a risk of complications. Hernia repair may be accomplished surgically using either open or laparoscopic techniques.

Accessible Repair:

Open hernia repair, also referred to as "herniorrhaphy" or "hernioplasty," is a conventional surgical technique in which the herniated tissue is accessed and repaired by creating an incision directly over the hernia site. To stop the projecting tissue from coming back, the weak abdominal wall is strengthened during the treatment using mesh or sutures.

Although open repair is popular and successful, it usually takes longer to recover from than laparoscopic repair and might cause greater pain after surgery. It is still a good choice, nevertheless, for certain individuals, especially those with more complicated or big hernias.

Laparoscopic Maintenance:

Known as "minimally invasive" or "keyhole" surgery, laparoscopic hernia repair entails creating many tiny abdominal incisions through which a laparoscope—a camera—and other specialized surgical devices are placed. Using mesh to bolster the weak spot, the surgeon repairs the hernia from inside the abdominal cavity using the camera and other tools.

When compared to open repair, laparoscopic repair has several potential advantages, such as shorter hospital stays, quicker recovery periods, and less discomfort after surgery. It could also lead to reduced scarring and a decreased chance of certain side effects, such as wound infections.

The decision between open and laparoscopic hernia repairs is based on several considerations, including the patient's overall health, and the size and location of the hernia, and both techniques are typically safe and successful. Healthcare professionals will talk about the various alternatives and, taking into account each patient's unique situation and preferences, suggest the best course of action.

People may cooperate with their healthcare professionals to make educated choices about their care and get the best results by being aware of the many hernia treatment alternatives. Long-term consequences may be avoided and quality of life enhanced by appropriately treating hernias, whether by surgical intervention, lifestyle modifications, or cautious waiting.

CHAPTER 5

Preparing For Surgery

Pre-Operative Instructions

It's vital to adhere to pre-operative instructions before hernia surgery to guarantee a seamless and safe procedure. Although your surgeon will give you particular advice based on your unique medical circumstances, certain basic suggestions are applicable in most situations.

First of all, before the procedure, you can be told to skip out on food and liquids for a certain amount of time. This is usually done to lower the possibility of issues during the surgery, such as aspiration—the inhalation of stomach contents into the lungs—while the patient is unconscious.

Apart from food limitations, your surgeon could advise you to abstain from taking certain drugs in the days before the procedure. These may include nonsteroidal anti-inflammatory medicines (NSAIDs) or blood thinners since they raise the possibility of bleeding during the surgery.

It's also crucial to let your surgeon know about any current medicines you use, including over-the-counter, prescription, and dietary supplements. To reduce risks, certain drugs may need to be changed or temporarily discontinued before surgery.

To assist lower the chance of infection at the surgical site, you may also be instructed to take a shower the night before or the morning of the procedure using a certain antibacterial soap. A good recovery depends on keeping the region sterile and bacterial-free.

Last but not least, on the day of the operation, make sure you have transportation to and from the hospital or surgical facility.

After anesthesia, you won't be able to drive yourself home, so it's crucial to have a friend or family member present to help you.

You may reduce the chance of problems and make sure you are well-prepared for hernia surgery by carefully adhering to these pre-operative guidelines.

What To Expect During Surgery

Usually, general anesthesia is used during hernia surgery, so you will be pain-free and unconscious the whole time. Your surgeon will create an incision close to the hernia location when anesthetized to reach the protruding tissue.

The kind and location of the hernia will determine the precise surgical approach. The protruding tissue is often pulled back into position, and to strengthen the weak abdominal wall and stop the hernia from happening again, a mesh or patch may be used.

Your surgeon will take great care throughout the surgery to minimize injury to the surrounding tissues and organs while repairing the hernia. After the repair is finished, surgical staples or stitches will be used to seal the wound.

Hernia surgery is often done as an outpatient operation, so when you've recovered from the anesthetic, you may return home that same day. However, in some complicated circumstances, post-operative care and supervision may need a brief hospital stay.

You could feel some pain or discomfort at the surgical site after the procedure, but your surgeon should be able to prescribe painkillers to help you deal with it. It's critical to adhere to your surgeon's post-operative care recommendations to facilitate recovery and lower the chance of problems.

Overall, hernia surgery has a high success rate and is a rather simple process. Knowing what to anticipate from surgery can help you go into the process with confidence and concentrate on getting well.

Potential Risks And Complications

Although hernia surgery is usually safe and successful, there are always some risks and consequences associated with any surgical operation. Before having surgery, it's important to be aware of these risks and to talk about them with your surgeon.

An infection at the operative site is one possible danger associated with hernia surgery. Your surgeon will use sterile equipment and antibiotics both before and after the surgery to reduce this risk. But it's crucial to keep an eye out for infection symptoms like redness, swelling, or discharge at the incision site, and to let your surgeon know as soon as you have any concerns.

Bleeding is another potential side effect of hernia surgery. Excessive bleeding during or after the surgery is rare but may happen. To reduce this risk, your surgeon will use techniques like cautery to close blood arteries during the process and refrain from taking blood thinners before the procedure.

Surgery to repair a hernia may sometimes cause harm to other organs or tissues, including blood arteries or nerves. The region around the surgery site may experience symptoms like numbness, tingling, or weakness as a result. Even though they are uncommon, you should address these problems with your physician before surgery.

Hernia recurrence is another possibility, particularly if the underlying cause of the hernia is not treated after surgery.

There is a little possibility that the hernia may reoccur in the future, but your surgeon will take precautions to strengthen the thin abdominal wall and lower the risk.

In general, the risks and consequences associated with hernia surgery are negligible, particularly when weighed against the possible advantages of healing the hernia and reducing symptoms. Assisting your surgeon in addressing your specific risk factors and closely adhering to pre-and post-operative instructions may reduce the probability of problems and lead to a favorable result.

CHAPTER 6

Recovery Process

Post-Operative Care Guidelines

A successful recovery after hernia repair surgery depends on receiving the right post-operative care. Here are some broad principles to follow, but your healthcare practitioner will offer specific advice based on your particular circumstances.

To avoid infection, the surgical site must be kept dry and clean. Your physician may advise using sterile dressings to keep the area dry and washing it gently with soap and water. To encourage healing and lower the risk of problems, make sure you carefully follow any advice about wound care.

Your doctor could also recommend drugs to treat pain and stop infections. It's important to take these drugs exactly as prescribed and to let your doctor know if you have any unexpected side effects or symptoms.

It's common to feel some soreness, swelling, and bruising at the surgery site during the first healing phase. By resting as much as you can and applying cold packs to the affected region for brief periods, you may help reduce these symptoms.

Maintaining a healthy diet is also crucial when recovering. For a while, your doctor may advise a soft or liquid food to facilitate digestion and lessen pressure on the surgery site. Solid meals may be gradually added back in as long as they're tolerated, but be sure to stay away from anything that might hurt or make your symptoms worse.

During this period, it is crucial to look after your mental health in addition to your physical healing. As having surgery may be a difficult event, don't hesitate to ask for emotional assistance from friends, family, or a support group.

Lastly, make sure you see your doctor for post-operative checkups on time. During these consultations, your doctor may assess any issues, keep an eye on your progress, and modify your treatment plan as needed.

By carefully adhering to these post-operative care instructions, you may prevent difficulties, encourage healing, and accelerate your recuperation.

Managing Pain And Discomfort

Following hernia repair surgery, pain and discomfort are typical, but there are a few helpful techniques to help manage these symptoms.

First, to aid with discomfort during the early stages of recuperation, your doctor can provide painkillers. It's important to take these drugs exactly as prescribed and to let your doctor know if you have any adverse effects or if your pain is not being well managed.

You may treat pain and discomfort using several non-pharmacological methods in addition to prescription drugs. Short-term use of ice packs at the surgical site may help numb the region, decrease swelling, and ease discomfort. Just be sure to cover the ice pack with a towel to avoid making direct skin contact, which may result in frostbite.

Deep breathing and relaxation techniques are also useful for alleviating pain. Deep breathing techniques may ease pain and accelerate recovery by assisting with muscle relaxation and tension reduction. Furthermore, methods like progressive muscle relaxation, guided visualization, and meditation may help divert your attention from the discomfort and foster a feeling of peace and well-being.

It's also crucial to adhere to your physician's advice on physical activity throughout the healing process. Gentle movement and mild exercise may help minimize stiffness and enhance circulation, which can benefit the healing process, even if it's crucial to relax and avoid intense activity immediately.

Lastly, make sure you discuss your pain thresholds and any worries you may have with your healthcare professional honestly and openly. Your physician can provide direction and encouragement to help you properly manage your pain and make a full recovery.

Resuming Normal Activities

You will progressively be able to return to your regular activities as you go through the healing process.

However, to prevent overexertion or injury, it's imperative that you go cautiously and pay attention to your body's signals.

When you can resume other activities, including driving, working out, and working out, your doctor will give you precise instructions. Carefully adhering to these instructions is necessary to avoid issues and encourage recovery.

To give your body time to recuperate correctly, you may need to take some time off from work at first. Depending on the sort of surgery you had and the specifics of your recuperation, your doctor will advise you on when it's safe to resume work.

In a similar vein, your doctor will advise you on when to start exercising and engaging in physical activity again. Exercise is vital to maintain circulation and avoid stiffness, but it's also important to start cautiously and build up to longer and more intense exercises as tolerated.

Waiting until you are no longer using prescription painkillers and can easily do all required motions, including braking and turning the steering wheel, is crucial when it comes to driving. Your doctor will offer you specialized advice based on your unique circumstances.

All things considered, the secret to getting back to your regular activities following hernia repair surgery is to pay attention to your body, do what your doctor advises, and gradually raise your activity level as tolerated. You may expedite the healing process, reduce difficulties, and return as soon as safely to your usual schedule by doing this.

CHAPTER 7

Complications And Recurrences

Possible Complications After Surgery

Although hernia repair surgery is usually safe, there are certain dangers involved, just as with any surgical operation. Being aware of these possible issues can help you plan and make wise choices.

Infection at the surgery site is one potential outcome. Even with the surgeon's greatest efforts to keep the area sterile, this may still happen. An infection manifests as redness, swelling, warmth, elevated discomfort, and pus coming out of the wound site. It's important to get in touch with your doctor right away if you see any of these symptoms since infections left untreated might worsen.

The hernia returning is another possible consequence. Hernias may sometimes recur even after successful treatment, particularly if the underlying problem that initially caused the hernia is left untreated. Risk factors for recurrence include obesity, strenuous lifting, and persistent coughing.

After surgery, some people could also have persistent discomfort. This may happen as a consequence of scar tissue development or nerve injury sustained during the surgery. While the body heals, this pain usually lessens with time for most people, it may not go away for others.

Hernia surgery may sometimes result in consequences including damage to nearby organs or blood vessels. While dangers are always there during surgery, surgeons take steps to reduce them.

Strategies To Prevent Hernia Recurrence

Even when surgery to fix a hernia is beneficial, it's crucial to take precautions against recurrence. Carefully adhering to your surgeon's recommendations throughout the healing phase will help avoid issues and enhance the procedure's long-term success.

Avoiding activities that exert tension on the surgical site during the first healing period is an important tactic. This usually entails avoiding intense activity and heavy lifting for a few weeks after surgery. You may contribute to a healthy result by allowing your body to mend without excessive stress.

A healthy weight and proper posture may also help lower the chance of a hernia recurrence. Being overweight increases the tension on the muscles in the abdomen, which raises the risk of developing or reoccurring an abdominal hernia.

Similarly, over time, bad posture may weaken the abdominal wall and increase its vulnerability to hernias.

Your surgeon may sometimes advise you to wear a supporting garment throughout the healing process, such as an abdominal binder. These clothes provide light compression to the surgical region, which may aid in healing and lessen edema.

Lastly, treating any underlying medical issues—like persistent coughing or constipation—that aided in the hernia's development will help avoid a recurrence. By managing these problems with your doctor, you may enhance your general health and lower your risk of developing hernias in the future.

When To Follow Up With Your Doctor

It's imperative that you schedule routine follow-up visits with your physician after hernia repair surgery.

These consultations provide your doctor the chance to track your healing process and spot any possible issues early on.

Generally speaking, two weeks after surgery is when you should make an appointment for a follow-up with your surgeon. Your surgeon will examine the location of your incision, evaluate the degree of your healing, and answer any queries or concerns you may have during this appointment.

Depending on your unique healing process, your doctor may suggest more visits after the first follow-up. Do not hesitate to call your doctor right away if you encounter any unexpected symptoms or consequences, such as increasing pain, swelling, or fever, in between consultations.

Sustained follow-up treatment is also necessary to monitor the effectiveness of the hernia repair and spot any recurrence warning indicators. To monitor your abdominal wall for any indications of weakening or a hernia recurrence, your doctor can advise routine examinations.

You may contribute to a good recovery and lower the chance of problems or recurrence by being proactive about your follow-up treatment and quickly addressing any issues.

CHAPTER 8

Living With A Hernia

Coping Strategies

Although having a hernia might be difficult, there are coping mechanisms that can be used to properly manage the disease. Recognizing your limits and not overdoing things are important. Avoiding exercises that put undue pressure on the abdominal muscles, including heavy lifting or vigorous activity, is crucial since they may make the hernia worse. Instead, concentrate on low-impact activities that build the muscles in the core without overstretching the injured region.

Wearing a supporting garment, such as a truss or hernia belt, to provide the weaker abdominal wall more support is another coping mechanism. These clothes may lessen pain and lower the possibility of hernia-related problems. Furthermore, keeping a healthy weight and adopting proper posture might help reduce discomfort and stop the hernia from becoming worse.

Furthermore, it's critical to pay attention to any warning signals or symptoms of problems, such as abrupt discomfort or swelling, and to listen to your body. Seeking immediate medical assistance if you encounter any worrisome symptoms will help guarantee appropriate hernia management and help avoid more severe problems.

It is essential to address the emotional burden of living with a hernia in addition to physical coping measures. The limits imposed by the illness might cause emotions of frustration, worry, or sadness in many people. Getting help from loved ones, friends, or a mental health professional may help you deal with these emotional difficulties and keep a positive perspective.

All things considered, a comprehensive strategy including social, mental, and physical coping mechanisms may assist people in properly managing and enduring a hernia while preserving their standard of living.

Diet And Exercise Recommendations

Exercise and diet are important factors in controlling a hernia and lowering the chance of complications. Dietary advice to avoid constipation, which may worsen hernia symptoms, should include meals that are simple to digest and rich in fiber. Your diet may encourage regular bowel movements and lessen the pressure on your abdominal muscles by including an abundance of fruits, vegetables, complete grains, and lean meats.

Constipation risk may be further decreased by remaining hydrated throughout the day by drinking plenty of water, which will assist soften and facilitate the passage of stools. Steer clear of meals heavy in fat, spice, or caffeine since these might aggravate the digestive tract and exacerbate the symptoms of a hernia.

Achieving a balance between exercise and avoiding activities that put undue tension on the abdominal muscles is crucial. Walking, swimming, and cycling are examples of low-impact workouts that may assist increase general fitness without placing too much strain on the hernia. Pilates and yoga are two forms of strengthening workouts that focus on the core muscles and may help support the abdominal wall.

However, it's important to stay away from hard lifting and high-impact exercises since they might exacerbate intra-abdominal pressure and aggravate the hernia. A physical therapist or medical expert may provide you with individualized advice based on your unique condition and degree of fitness if you're not sure whether activities are safe for you.

Incorporating low-impact exercise and maintaining a balanced diet will help manage your hernia while also enhancing your general health and well-being.

Psychological Impact And Support Resources

The psychological effects of having a hernia may be profound, impairing a person's quality of life and mental stability. Many may feel depressed, frustrated, or anxious as they deal with the difficulties brought on by the illness. To guarantee comprehensive therapy for the hernia, it is important to identify and address these emotional problems.

Dealing with the emotional effects of having a hernia may be made easier by asking for help from friends, family, or a mental health professional. Open communication about your emotions and worries may reduce tension and give you a sense of relaxation. Joining online forums or support groups for people with hernias may also provide helpful peer support and helpful information for managing the illness.

Apart from providing emotional support, obtaining trustworthy information and resources on hernias may enable people to actively participate in the management of their disease. Healthcare providers, including physicians and nurses, may provide direction and information on available treatments, coping mechanisms, and lifestyle adjustments to enhance the management of hernias.

Additionally, being up to date on the most recent developments in hernia research and treatment may assist patients in making well-informed choices about their care. Those looking to learn more about hernias and the available treatments may find a wealth of information by visiting websites, reading books, and contacting respectable medical associations.

By addressing the psychological effects of having a hernia and getting access to the right kind of assistance, people may improve their quality of life and general well-being while managing the disease.

CHAPTER 9

Hernia In Special Populations

Hernias In Infants And Children

First of all, hernias, which are often seen as bulges in the abdominal wall due to a weakness in the muscle or tissue, are a frequent condition in babies and toddlers. Treat them right immediately to avoid repercussions, even if they may not ache all the time.

Different Types of Young People's Hernias:

1. Inguinal hernias are the most common kind of hernia in newborns and children. When a portion of the intestine protrudes via a weak spot in the abdominal muscles, it causes a protrusion in the labia in females and the groin or scrotum in boys.

2. Umbilical Hernias: These occur as a protrusion at the navel and are also very prevalent. They appear when some intestinal or abdominal lining protrudes after childbirth due to a weakening of the muscles protecting the belly button.

Diagnosis and Treatment:

A physical examination is often used by a medical professional to identify hernias in newborns and children. Sometimes the diagnosis may be verified with ultrasounds and other imaging testing.

In this age bracket, treating hernias usually involves surgery. Specifically, inguinal hernias are usually surgically corrected to prevent problems such as incarceration or strangulation, which may occur when the herniated tissue gets trapped and the blood supply is interrupted.

Fortunately, hernia repair surgery for infants and children is often safe and effective. The majority of kids recover from the surgery with little to no problems. To guarantee a speedy recovery, parents must, however, go by the post-operative care guidelines given by the medical staff.

Hernias During Pregnancy

First off, because of the increased strain on the abdominal and pelvic area as the baby develops, pregnancy may sometimes worsen or even cause hernias in women. Although hernias are not common in pregnant women, it is important to recognize the warning signs and symptoms.

Various Kinds of Hernias During Gestation:

1. Umbilical hernias: As the uterus grows, pregnant women may acquire new umbilical hernias or observe that pre-existing ones become more noticeable, placing extra pressure on the abdominal muscles.

2. Inguinal Hernias: These are less prevalent during pregnancy, but they may still happen, particularly in women who have had stomach surgery or prior pregnancies.

Diagnosis and Management: Pregnancy-related hernias are often diagnosed by a physical examination performed by a healthcare professional. To minimize any difficulties, surgery to treat the hernia is usually postponed until after birth, however, it may be advised in some circumstances.

Relieving symptoms and reducing pain are often the main goals of managing hernias during pregnancy. This might include keeping proper posture, refraining from hard lifting or straining, and using supporting clothing.

Postpartum Care: Following childbirth, postpartum care is essential for women undergoing hernia repair surgery. Maintaining wound care, limiting physical activity, and scheduling follow-up visits to the healthcare provider's recommendations help promote appropriate healing and reduce the likelihood of problems.

Hernias In Older Adults

First of all, the weakening of the abdominal muscles and tissues with age raises the incidence of hernias. Elderly people who cough a lot, are obese, or have had prior surgery may also be more susceptible to hernias.

Different Types of Hernias in Seniors:

1. Inguinal Hernias: These continue to be the most prevalent kind of hernia among the elderly, often manifesting as bulges in the groin region.

They may cause pain in the pelvic area in women and spread into the scrotum in males.

2. Incisional Hernias: These are conditions where tissue protrudes through the site of a prior surgical incision and are common in older persons who have had abdominal procedures in the past.

Diagnose and Therapy: Just as in other age groups, the diagnosis of hernias in older persons usually entails a physical examination by a medical professional. To quantify the extent of the hernia and confirm the diagnosis, imaging investigations like CT or ultrasound may be carried out.

Surgery is usually required to repair hernias in older adults, especially if the hernia is causing symptoms or issues like intestinal obstruction or strangulation. When possible, minimally invasive techniques might be carried out to reduce recovery time and suffering after surgery.

Postoperative Care and Recovery: Due to factors including reduced mobility and delayed healing, older people may need longer recovery times after hernia repair surgery than younger people. On the other hand, according to the physician's orders for wound care, activity restrictions, and rehabilitation exercises may help to maximize healing and lower the risk of recurrence.

CHAPTER 10

Future Directions In Hernia Management

Emerging Treatments And Technologies

New medications and technologies provide exciting opportunities for improved patient outcomes and rehabilitation in the constantly changing field of hernia treatment. The use of less intrusive techniques like laparoscopic and robotically assisted surgery is one significant advancement. Compared to traditional open surgeries, these methods include fewer incisions, less tissue stress, and quicker recovery times. Many find minimally invasive hernia surgery to be an enticing option since patients often have less postoperative pain and may resume normal activities sooner.

The use of biological meshes in hernia therapy is another encouraging development. Biologic meshes are made from human or animal tissue and gradually absorbed by the body over time, in contrast to ordinary synthetic meshes that remain in the body indefinitely. This characteristic reduces the likelihood of chronic issues like recurrent pain and infections linked to the mesh. Additionally, biological meshes may promote tissue remodeling and in growth, which would improve the outcomes of hernia repair.

Furthermore, advancements in imaging technologies have enabled improvements in preoperative planning and intraoperative navigation. Thanks to high-resolution imaging technology like CT and MRI scans, surgeons may accurately evaluate a hernia's size, location, and characteristics before treating it. During surgery, real-time imaging techniques like intraoperative ultrasonography help to guide the placement of the mesh and guarantee the best possible repair.

Research Advancements

Long-term studies of the treatment of hernias have produced significant advances in our understanding of the underlying pathophysiology, risk factors, and treatment strategies. One area of research is the role that genetics plays in the development and recurrence of hernias. Scientists want to develop customized therapy regimens that consider the distinct genetic profiles of individual patients by identifying genetic markers associated with an increased risk of hernias.

Current clinical trials are investigating novel surgical techniques, implant materials, and postoperative care instructions to further enhance the outcomes of hernia repairs. For example, studies on the efficacy of tissue engineering techniques seek to develop bioengineered scaffolds that promote tissue regeneration and lower the risk of recurrence. Likewise, research on enhanced pain management strategies seeks to lessen surgical discomfort and increase patient contentment.

Furthermore, advancements in biomaterial science have led to the creation of next-generation meshes with improved biocompatibility and biomechanical characteristics. These innovative materials aim to reduce the possibility of mesh-related issues including migration, shrinkage, and fibrosis by providing enough support for tissue recovery. In light of the most current scientific discoveries, researchers strive to enhance the long-term outcomes for hernia patients by consistently refining surgical techniques and implant materials.

Patient Advocacy And Support Groups

In addition to medical advancements, patient advocacy, and support groups are crucial for empowering individuals with hernias and their families. These organizations provide useful resources, information, and emotional support to patients as they navigate the route from hernia diagnosis to recovery.

Participating in a hernia support group provides an opportunity to talk with others who have experienced similar situations and share advice and experiences. One of the key benefits is this. Peer support may be very beneficial in lowering the anxiety and feelings of loneliness that are often associated with the diagnosis and treatment of hernias. Patients who participate in online forums, local support groups, and educational events may exchange experiences, gain understanding from one another's viewpoints, and find solace in knowing that they are not alone in their recovery journey.

Furthermore, patient advocacy groups play a critical role in educating the public about hernias and advocating for improved access to high-quality care and treatment options. These organizations work to close gaps in the system and advocate legislation that prioritizes patient safety and well-being via collaborations with lawmakers, healthcare professionals, and business leaders.

Furthermore, patient advocacy groups are often a fantastic resource for patient education and empowerment, providing them with the knowledge and tools they need to make informed healthcare decisions. These groups aim to empower hernia sufferers to take control of their condition and act as advocates for their health and welfare. They do this by providing webinars, instructional materials, insurance coverage guidance, and financial aid initiatives.

Future developments in the area of hernia care should bring improved outcomes and a higher quality of life for patients worldwide. These may be accomplished by putting new treatments and technological advancements to good use, encouraging research initiatives, and setting up patient advocacy and support groups.

CONCLUSION

To sum up, hernias are a significant medical condition that needs careful attention and treatment. With an increased understanding of hernias throughout time, advances in diagnosis, treatment, and prevention have been made. From ancient times, when hernias were believed to be caused by gods, to the present, when we have sophisticated surgical techniques and a thorough grasp of anatomy, it has been an incredible journey.

In contemporary medicine, hernias may be repaired using a variety of techniques, including open surgery, laparoscopic procedures, and robotically assisted surgeries. There are advantages and disadvantages to each procedure, and the choice depends on several factors, including the patient's health, the surgeon's expertise, and the kind and size of the hernia.

It is important to recognize the potential complications resulting from hernias, such as intestinal obstruction, asphyxia, and incarceration. Neglecting to handle these problems might have serious consequences. Therefore, quick intervention is required to prevent issues and improve patient outcomes.

Furthermore, taking preventive action is largely responsible for avoiding hernias. Hernia risk may be decreased by changing lifestyle habits to include things like maintaining a healthy weight, avoiding heavy lifting, and utilizing the proper lifting techniques, especially in people with risk factors like obesity or a chronic cough.

In addition to surgery, ongoing research aims to explore alternative treatment strategies and improve our understanding of the pathophysiology of hernias. Our objective is to improve treatment strategies for hernias and improve patients' outcomes over the long term by looking at genetic predispositions, tissue biomechanics, and biomaterial developments.

In conclusion, although hernias provide challenges, they also serve as a testament to the persistence and creativity of medical science. With an emphasis on early detection, prevention, and effective treatment, we continue to advance the comprehensive care of hernias via interdisciplinary collaboration, technology advancements, and a patient-centered approach.

THE END

www.ingramcontent.com/pod-product-compliance
Lightning Source LLC
Chambersburg PA
CBHW061258250726
48653CB00002B/679